The Migraine Diet
Cut the Additives & Clear the Toxins

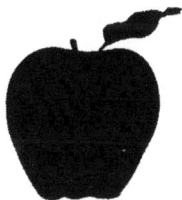

by J. Corne

The Migraine Diet
Cut the Additives & Clear the Toxins

By J Corne

Original Copyright 2008,

All Rights Reserved

J Corne

Edited and Reformatted, 2016

Table of Contents

This book was written as a result of my personal health struggle with migraine disorder.

It is not intended for diagnoses or definitive treatment of migraine or other physical conditions; I am not a physician.

I follow The Migraine Diet and utilize prophylactic medication to control migraine and hope this information will be a useful tool for you in reducing the frequency & severity of migraines and improving your overall health.

Good luck.

-J Corne

Migraine: Why is This Happening?

Migraine is typically described as a condition with symptoms that include headache (characterized by throbbing pain usually on one side of the head); aura (visual disturbances); nausea and vomiting; sensitivity to lights, sounds, smells or movement; dizziness; difficulty concentrating; and diarrhea. In rare cases those experiencing a migraine may suffer weakness, language difficulties or other neurological disorders. Migraines are typically believed to last from 4-72 hours and disrupt regular activities or prevent all activity during that time.

For many years, scientists believed that migraines were linked to the dilation and constriction of blood vessels in the head. Researchers [now] believe that migraine is the result of fundamental neurological abnormalities caused by genetic mutations at work in the brain.

At the height of my own migraine struggles, I was hospitalized because the symptoms I experienced so closely resembled stroke, disrupted vision, numb limbs (specifically the left arm), confusion and difficulty with speech. These were replaced by unbearable head pain and uncontrollable vomiting.

In my late twenties, as migraines became more disruptive and severe in my life, I became desperate and began to seek answers as I wondered, "Why is this happening to me?" I was surprised again and again by the tepid answers I received from my general physician and the neurologists I visited.

At my most pessimistic, I interpreted their lack of treatment information as disinterest, but what I have more subjectively come to understand is that the causes of migraine are so varied that it is difficult to tell any one person exactly what to do to make them stop. "How do we treat this condition?" was my next question and initially, I didn't know enough about it to trust my own judgments. I was run through a trial of tests and medications that had little or no effect on the frequency and severity of the increasingly common migraines I suffered and I was given a list of 'commonly cited migraine triggers' to avoid. Diet specific information was delivered with a wave of the hand and disclaimed with "…**scientific evidence supporting a link between diet and migraine is largely anecdotal** ". Years ago, I believed this to mean my diet could not affect, positively or negatively, the frequency or intensity of the migraines I suffered. I look back now and think *how could I have been so wrong*?

And though food may not be a migraine trigger for all sufferers, if you are at the end-of-the-line in seeking avenues toward reducing the frequency and severity of migraine you may find it worthwhile to seriously consider diet change and its potential for positive outcome.

~

What's in our food? What's in *your* food?

Finding the right foods to fuel our bodies is not simple. We have so many options it's easy to become overwhelmed. Our choices are based enormously on what has been marketed to us, and supermarket shelves are loaded with foods that are colored, flavored, scented and preserved to give us easy, beautiful meals or desserts in the blink of an eye. Our emotions tell us go! The price tells us go! And the promise of a quicker, easier, more fabulous lifestyle tells us Go! Go! Go! When will we stop? When will we take the time to look around and ask the food manufacturers what's going into all of these colored, flavored, scented and preserved foods? Do we really need them? And what do they do to our bodies?

When *I* stopped and looked around, I started to ask some of these questions, and when I became aware of all the additives and preservatives in our food, I realized that what I put into my body *would* affect my

health and my diet *could* affect, positively or

negatively, the frequency and intensity of the migraines I suffered.

As I was having little luck at the time with prescriptive medications, I began to carefully observe my food intake & lifestyle decisions and how each affected my health. Through this observation, reading and research I went out on a limb and determined that the migraines I suffered might be the result of an inefficient processing of toxins in my body.

What I learned is surprising and although the lists of additives, preservatives and toxins I have compiled in this book seems daunting, I have found it has been possible to modify my diet to cut out some, many, then nearly all that are troublesome for me. **It is impossible to cut out all additives and preservatives from my diet and still have something to eat,** but it *is* possible to eat a healthy diet that is *relatively* free of additives & preservatives.

For me, the commitment, patience and time required

to prepare freshly made, carefully selected (additive & preservative free) foods has been well worthwhile; I have experienced a reduction in the frequency and severity of migraines.

~

"Commonly Cited" Migraine Triggers

Many health professionals offer a list of "Common Migraine Triggers" to their migraine patients. The basic list includes MSG, Red Wine, Chocolate and Cheese. This list is too short, incomplete and entirely too vague for the following reasons.

1. MSG (Monosodium Glutamate) is not always listed as such on food labels. It has many names that give no suggestion of its real identity; package label claims of 'NO MSG' can therefore never be trusted.

2. Red wine is almost always singled out as the alcoholic culprit in triggering migraines. This is very likely due to the presence of naturally occurring sulphites in red wine as well as the use of tannins and fermentation in its preparation. Overlooked is the fact that tannins are used to clarify both wine and beer and all alcohols are fermented during preparation, therefore making them all suspect as migraine triggers.

3. Chocolate has been linked to migraine because it is known to contain a compound known as tyramine. Research however has been inconclusive in determining whether or not the amount of tyramine in chocolate is adequate to trigger a migraine. It may be that a good quality chocolate with minimal ingredients (in moderation) is not a bad thing. Instead, cheap chocolates with additives and fillers could be the culprit in triggering 'chocolate migraines".

4. Cheese. As there are many varieties and preparations of cheese, it is helpful to be specific about which kinds of cheeses may act as migraine triggers. Aged cheeses (like emmental and parmesan), whey products and cheeses with flavorings & additives are potential migraine triggers due to their high tyramine content (in the aged &

whey products) or additives (as in the flavored products). Moderate amounts of soft cheeses like mozzarella and goat cheese may pose no trigger threat.

~

Toxins & Neurotoxins

The word '**toxin**' has many definitions. Essentially, a toxin is a poisonous substance produced by a living organism that is harmful to other cells, organisms or the body. Toxic substances of non-biological origin are called poisons and in the context of alternative medicine, 'toxin' is often used to refer to any substance claimed to cause illness or poor health.

As migraines are believed to be a neurological disorder, it is important to note *neurotoxins* as toxins that act specifically on nerve cells of the nervous system. This would include cells of the brain and spinal cord and all nerves extending to other areas of the body.

12

Neurotoxicity can occur when exposure to toxic substances or poisons affects the normal activity of the nervous system by disrupting or damaging neurons, the key cells that transmit and process signals from the brain and other parts of the nervous system. Exposure to certain foods, food additives, pesticides, cleaning solvents and cosmetics are often cited as potential hazards for individuals vulnerable to neurotoxins.

Additives

Monosodium Glutamate (MSG)

MSG appears to be the most common food additive and flavor enhancer in our food supply today. It is produced by the fermentation of starch and sugar and is sometimes labeled as a 'natural' product. Monosodium Glutamate is a well known migraine trigger that is often hidden in ingredient lists under names other than its own. It is found in most of the processed foods on our supermarket shelves today, in items such as canned soups, stock mixes, seasoning mixes, snack foods and fast foods.

The toxicity of Monosodium Glutamate has been studied since the early 1950s to today and the discovery by researcher John Olney in 1969 of the destructive effects of MSG on the brain cells of mice led him to coin the term **excitotoxicity** which is, "the pathological process by which nerve cells are damaged and killed by glutamate and similar substances."

Excitotoxicity has recently been tentatively linked to migraine in new research and medical hypotheses. In my experience, cutting 'excitotoxic additives' from my diet has made a world of difference in reducing the severity and frequency of migraines. Following is a list of some of the 'hidden names' of MSG.

Avoiding MSG (the hidden names of Monosodium Glutamate)

The following additives always contain MSG

Hydrolyzed Protein (plant, vegetable, any kind), Autolyzed Plant Protein, Vegetable Protein Extract, Sodium Casseinate, Calcium Casseinate,

Autolyzed Yeast, Yeast Extract, Yeast Food, Yeast Nutrient, Textured Protein, Glutamic Acid, Monopotassium Glutamate, Gelatin

May contain or create MSG during processing

Natural Flavors, flavoring, flavors, natural 'anything' flavor, Artificial Flavor, Bouillon or Stock, Broth (chicken, beef, vegetable, any kind), Carrageenan, Whey Protein, Whey Protein Concentrate, Whey Protein Isolate, Wheat Protein, Rice Protein, Corn Protein, Oat Protein, Protein Powders (as in protein bars, shakes and body building drinks), Rice Syrup, Cornstarch Fructose, Corn Syrup, Corn Syrup Solids, High Fructose Corn Syrup, Citric Acid (when processed from corn), Milk Powder, Dry Milk Solids, Annatto, Soy Sauce, Soy Protein Isolate, Soy Protein Concentrate, Malt Extract or Flavoring, Malted Barley, Maltodextrin, Dextrose, Dextrates, Gums (guar and vegetable), Dough Conditioners, Caramel Flavoring / Coloring, Pectin, Protease, Protease enzymes, Lecithin, Amino Acids (as in liquid amino acids), Flowing Agents, anything Enriched or Vitamin Enriched, anything Protein

Fortified, anything Fermented, anything Ultra Pasteurized, anything Enzyme-Modified

Another well known migraine trigger that is an Excitotoxic Additive is Aspartame. Aspartame is known to cause neural tissue damage in rodents.

Why Are Additives Used?

Additives are used for numerous reasons; whether they are necessary or beneficial in all cases is questionable. They are used for flavor enhancement, to slow spoilage, improve nutritional value and to simplify large scale product preparation.

The Food and Drug Administration (FDA) in the United States monitors food and drug products entering the consumer market with a mission to "…promote and protect the public health by helping safe and effective products reach the market in a timely way, to monitor products for continued safety after they are in use, and to help the public get the accurate, science-based information needed to improve health". In 1958, the Food Additives Amendment required scientific testing on all chemicals intentionally added to food. At this time the FDA established the GRAS (Generally Recognized As Safe) list for foods that were *assumed* to be safe for consumption and included additives such as sugar, starch, salt and baking soda. These were not tested for toxicity or safety and some GRAS items have since been found unsafe. Additives that remain on the GRAS list today that may be questionable for our safety and may be recognized as toxins in our bodies are shown in the following list. The potential health risks posed by these additives range from gastric irritation and asthmatic & allergic reactions to weakened immune systems and tumors.

GRAS Additives That May Be Unsafe *(not a complete list)*

Acacia Gum (Gum Arabic)
Commonly found in: gum, hard/soft candies, frostings

Chondrus Extract (Carrageenan)

Commonly found in: creamy, frozen and cheese foods

Tragacanth

Commonly found in: dressings, fruit sherbets & jellies

Carob or Locust Bean Gum

Commonly found in: gelatin desserts, ice cream

Alginic Acid (all alginates)

Commonly found in: creamy, frozen foods, spreads and dressings

Benzoic Acid/Sodium Benzoate

Commonly found in: soft drinks, fruit drinks, jams/jellies, margarine, pickles, beer, canned fruit

BHA/BHT

Commonly found in: breakfast cereals, dry mixes, instant mixes, candy, gum, shortening

Iron Salts (ferrous or ferric...)

Commonly found in: enriched breads, breakfast cereals, self-rising flour, cornmeal

Saccharin

Commonly found in: soft drinks

Sulphites

Commonly found in: almost anything fresh, dried, canned or processed

Nitrites & Nitrates

Commonly found in: processed meats

~

Sulphites

Sulphites (also spelled 'sulfites') have been banned in the United States, from use on food that is intended to be eaten raw. Unfortunately, their use may continue because of their efficiency as sanitary agents and preservatives for fresh produce. People who are prone to allergies or are asthmatic or deficient in the liver enzyme sulphite oxidase are warned of the dangers of sulphites as potentially lethal and they are often cited as a trigger for migraine sufferers. Sulphites are extremely common. They are not always listed with food ingredient information; especially on items where they are naturally present (i.e. wine & some vinegars).If listed on food ingredient lists, sulphites will be labeled under one of the following names:

Sodium Sulphite, Sulphur Dioxide, Sodium Bisulphite, Sodium Metabisulphate, Potassium Bisulphate, Potassium Metabisulphate

Sulphites are found in most processed products including:

precut potato products, french fries, hash browns, cookies, crackers, crusts, tortillas, breads, bottled and canned drinks, candy, syrups, gelatin, canned soups, stews, fish, meat, canned fruits and vegetables, condiments, salad dressings, mixes, cornstarch, drugs, dried fruits and other 'preserved' foods.

Nitrites

Nitrites are also used frequently in food processing today. They are used in combination with other additives during the curing of meats to delay spoilage and create a desired dark red 'cured-meat' color. They are highly toxic. "The lethal dose [of nitrites] for humans is approximately 22mg per kg/body weight" and they are known to form nitrosamines, (a potent cancer-causing substance) when reacting with the natural chemicals of our bodies.

~

Caffeine

Caffeine is a psychoactive drug. It acts as a stimulant on the central nervous & respiratory systems and heart and can cause nervousness, insomnia and irregular heartbeat. It may trigger migraine by causing lack of sleep, dehydration or elevated blood pressure. It is a vaso-constrictor which causes blood vessels to constrict, and then expand into painful spasms. Caffeine is found naturally in coffee, tea and chocolate and as an additive in many soft drinks and drugs.

Is Decaf the Right Choice?

Choosing decaffeinated coffee over caffeinated varieties may not always be the right choice.

Methylene chloride, which was commonly used as a caffeine solvent for seventy years before the 1980s was found at that time to have carcinogenic properties and its use was abandoned by many large U.S. coffee companies.

The FDA however, continues to allow manufacturers to utilize methylene chloride if the residues in the coffee are below 10 parts per million. Depending on the amount and type of decaffeinated coffee you drink and your sensitivity to methylene chloride residue, this may or may not pose a problem as a migraine trigger.

Swiss Water Decaffeinated coffees may be a worthy option if you love coffee but not the caffeine and manufacturing residues.

~

Vitamin Supplements & Medication

I avoid unnecessary vitamin supplements and medications and look very carefully at the labels of those I intend to use. Most contain a long list of non-medicinal additives, flavors and sugars.

Further, the possibility of rebound-headache due to over-use of analgesic medication provides good reason to avoid pain killer and other over-the-counter pain remedies.

Sample Supplement Ingredient List

Additives and ingredients suspect as migraine triggers are highlighted in **bold** print below,

Common Daily Vitamin Supplement / *In addition to vitamin and mineral content, non-medicinal ingredients are:* ***acacia, ascorbic palmitate, butylated hydroxytoluene, calcium silicate, cellulose, croscarmellose, sodium dextrin, dextrose, FD & C blue #2, yellow #5 and #6, gelatin, hypromellose, lecithin, magnesium stearate, partially hydrogenated soybean oil,*** *polyethylene glycol, resin, silicon dioxide, sodium carboxymethylcellellose, sodium citrate dihydrate, sodium lauryl sulphate,* starch, *stearic acid, sucrose, titanium dioxide.*

~

Food Labels That Mislead

Some labels do not provide clear facts about the products they contain as indicated by the following examples:

No Artificial Flavors

Foods labeled with this claim can still contain 'natural flavors' which are naturally occurring chemicals that may contain substances such as MSG (monosodium glutamate) and HVP (hydrolyzed vegetable protein).

No Preservatives

Items can be labeled 'No Preservatives' but still contain preservatives as part of the ingredients the manufacturer bought *to create the product*. They can also contain *artificial* colors and *Additives* with this label.

Naturally Sweetened

'Natural' has no legal FDA definition. This could mean the product is sweetened by any undefined 'natural' (remember, this term has no legal FDA definition) chemical process.

Natural or All Natural

The term 'natural' may refer to only specific ingredients and does not guarantee the product as a whole is free of additives and preservatives. Also, as mentioned 'natural' has no legal FDA definition.

Organic

Processed foods labeled 'made with organic ingredients' can still contain additives and chemicals, notably MSG and products that contain MSG.

*Special note on poultry When buying poultry certified 'organic', this label (often) means specifically the birds are from farms that meet standards mandating the use of organic feed, prohibiting the use of antibiotics and requiring the animals have fresh air and sunlight.

There is no mention in USDA Regulation Marketing literature regarding treatment after slaughter so it is important to be aware that during normal (non-organic) meat/poultry processing, meats and poultry are commonly soaked in or 'pumped' with hydrolyzed proteins (or other preservatives) to maintain freshness and improve taste. Smaller producers and farmers who can deliver fresh products quickly may not take this step in processing. Whether or not the 'organic' label means preservatives have not been used during processing is unclear.

When buying, it takes a lot of time and effort to discover the truth about how poultry and meat have been processed. Treating animal products with preservatives and chemicals has become so commonplace today, it seems many producers have almost forgotten they do it and are therefore entirely unprepared to be questioned about it.

~

Organic and Natural Do Not Always Mean Good For You.

I have encountered one or two well-meaning acquaintances who have become frustrated when I decline their 'healthy' organic meal offerings because of questionable additives.

Organic/natural soup broths for example, often contain Yeast Extract (albeit organic), Natural Flavorings and Gums. Organic/natural chips very often contain Maltodextrin, Dextrose and Natural Flavors; all of which are included on the list of 'hidden names of MSG'.

~

Sample Ingredient Lists

'Diet' Foods

Before I began my search for a healthier diet that would help in the management of migraines, I assumed that 'diet' foods or foods labeled as 'healthy choices' would improve my health. I could not have been further from the truth. One look at the exceedingly long list of ingredients on the prepackaged diet foods in the supermarket will tell you just how 'good' they are. 'Health' symbols are not always a guarantee that what you are getting is healthy. The following is a sample of the ingredients from one such package. Additives and ingredients suspect as migraine triggers are highlighted in **bold** print.

Frozen 'Diet' Dinner with special notation of 'No Preservatives'/ Ingredients: cooked noodles (water, semolina, wheat gluten), **cooked seasoned chicken (chicken breast meat, glaze** *[water,* **seasoning, (modified corn starch,** *salt, dehydrated garlic,* **spices,** *dehydrated onion,* **citric acid,** *dehydrated parsley); canola oil,* **maltodextrin, caramel color***], water, modified potato starch,* **soy protein isolate, chicken flavor [autolyzed yeast extract,** *salt,* **soy sauce (soy beans,** *wheat, salt), sugar,* **maltodextrin,** *dehydrated chicken,* **flavor,** *sesame oil,* **dehydrated chicken broth, lactic acid, citric acid,** *chicken fat],* **sodium phosphates,** *water, yellow zucchini, zucchini,* **milk ingredients,**

parmesan cheese, soy oil, *onions*, **modified corn starch**, *salt, garlic, onion powder*, **potassium chloride**, *rice starch*, **autolyzed yeast extract**, *sugar*, **spices, carrageenan, color, dextrose, flavor (salt, autolyzed yeast extract, maltodextrin, flavor, chicken powder, soy sauce [soy bean**, *wheat, salt*], **milk ingredients**.

Common Supermarket Foods

Below are the ingredient lists of 11 common supermarket foods; some are labeled as 'healthy' or 'smart', others are labeled in a way that might lead you to believe you are eating something that is healthier for you than it really is. Note the length of the ingredient lists and how many additives there are. Additives and ingredients suspect as migraine triggers are highlighted in **bold** print.

Breakfast Cereal with 'Health Check' symbol from the Heart and Stroke Foundation/ Ingredients: whole grain oats, **modified corn starch, corn starch**, *sugar, salt*, **trisodium phosphate, calcium carbonate, monoglycerides, annatto,**

tocopherols, *wheat starch.*

Flavoured Instant Oatmeal with special notation of 'No Artificial Colors'/ Ingredients: rolled oats, sugar, **guar gum, modified milk ingredients**, *salt,* **natural and artificial flavor, calcium carbonate (thickener), caramel color (contains sulphites**), *wheat starch, silicon dioxide, vitamins and minerals [iron, niacinamide, zinc oxide, thiamine mononitrate, calcium pantothenate, pyridoxine hydrochloride (vitamin B6), folic acid].*

Fat Free Yogurt/ Ingredients: skim milk, strawberries, **concentrated skim milk**, *peaches, sugar,* **fructose, corn starch, milk protein concentrate**, *cream,* **modified corn starch, gelatin**, *active bacterial cultures,* **natural flavors, sodium citrate, natural colors, (annatto**: *peach)* (**carmine**: *strawberry),* **malic acid, potassium sorbate**, *vitamin A palmitate, vitamin D; made with vitamin A & D fortified skim milk.*

*Canned Soup/ Ingredients: chicken broth, rice***,** **seasoned chicken**, *carrots, salt, chicken fat, potato* starch, water, celery, **monosodium glutamate, chicken flavor, mechanically separated chicken meat**, dehydrated onions, **spice,** beta carotene, **disodium guanylate, disodium inosinate, soy protein isolate,** dehydrated garlic and **lactic acid.**

'Healthy' Canned Soup with 'Health Check' symbol from the Heart and Stroke Foundation/ Ingredients: beef broth, (water, **beef stock**) carrots, potatoes, tomato paste, **seasoned beef**, celery, diced tomatoes **(tomatoes, tomato juice, citric acid, calcium chloride**), green beans, peas, **corn,** barley, potato starch, **beef flavor, enriched wheat flour**, dehydrated onions, **hydrolyzed yeast protein, yeast extract and hydrolyzed wheat gluten, modified corn starch**, sugar, **potassium chloride,** salt, dehydrated garlic, **caramel, spice**, sea salt and parsley.

Low Fat Peanut Butter/ Ingredients: roasted peanuts, **maltodextrin**, sugar, salt, hydrogenated vegetable oil

Organic Snack Food with special notation indicating

"No Artificial Flavors or Colors"/ Ingredients:
organic potatoes, organic sunflower oil, **organic**
seasoning (organic corn maltodextrin, organic
spices*, sea salt,* **organic dextrose, silicon**
dioxide, natural flavor*, organic sunflower oil,* **citric**
acid*, sea salt.*

Snack Food with special notation indicating "No
Artificial Flavors or Colors"/ Ingredients: popcorn,
canola and/or sunflower oil, **white cheddar cheese**
seasoning (modified milk ingredients, white
cheddar cheese solids, maltodextrin*, salt,*
*sunflower oil***, corn syrup solids, sugar, modified**
corn starch, disodium phosphate, blue cheese
solids, lactic acid, citric acid, dipotassium
phosphate, mono-and diglycerides, soy lecithin,
hydroxylated soy lecithin, natural flavor, l-
glutamic acid, calcium silicate, silicon dioxide*).*

Low Fat Snack Food with special notation indicating
"No Artificial Flavors or Colors"/ Ingredients: rice,
yellow corn flour, **seasoning** *[sugar, salt,*
maltodextrin, natural flavor*, (including* **wasabi**
flavor*),* **soya sauce powder** *(wheat,* **soybeans),**

honey powder, spices, *wheat starch, sunflower oil, onion powder***, malic acid, hydroxylated soy lecithin**, *turmeric***, calcium silicate, calcium stearate***], high oleic safflower oil, sea salt.*

Frozen Chicken Fingers with special note of '0 Trans Fat'/ Ingredients: **chicken breast** *(may contain traces of egg), water,* **modified milk ingredients, soy protein (contains soy lecithin)**, *salt, garlic powder,* **spices in a breading** *of: water, wheat flour, toasted wheat crumbs***, cornstarch, modified cornstarch**, *yellow corn flour, salt, sugar***, soy protein, spices, dextrose**, *onion powder,* **sodium aluminum phosphate, sodium bicarbonate, autolyzed yeast extract, flavor**, *browned in canola oil.*

Chocolate Bar/ Ingredients: sugar, wafer (sugar, vegetable oil, modified palm kernel oil, wheat flour, **cornstarch, soy lecithin**, *salt, sodium bicarbonate***, citric acid, artificial flavor***) **glucose-fructose**, *modified palm oil, modified vegetable oil***, modified milk ingredients, crisped rice** *(rice, sugar, salt***, malt flavor** *(wheat)), unsweetened chocolate,* *glucose syrup*, *peanuts, cocoa butter*, **soy lecithin**, *salt*, **citric acid, natural flavor.**

~

Amines

Of the huge number of additives discussed thus far, the most notable decrease in the frequency and severity of my migraines occurred when I cut out MSG, hydrolyzed products, meats with nitrites, protein additives, malt, cornstarch, corn syrup, and chewing gums. Food Additives seem to be my greatest migraine trigger but it is also important to note a naturally occurring family of protein components called amines, which have been linked to migraine.

The Amines:

Dopamine
Commonly found in: peanuts, peas, broad beans, soy

Tyramine

Commonly found in: aged foods such as hard cheeses, yogurt, buttermilk, wine, fresh produce that is deteriorating (over-ripe) and fermented foods

Histamine

Commonly found in: coldwater fish such as salmon and tuna

Phenyl ethylamine

Commonly found in: chocolate

Octopamine

Commonly found in: citrus

Tryptamine

Commonly found in: tomatoes and pineapple

Detoxification

As my diet research continued, I came to a point when I had gathered enough information to realize that a serious change in my eating habits would help in decreasing the frequency and severity of migraines. I wanted to change my diet and kick-started the change by getting rid of whatever toxins had already built up inside of me.

A Detoxification Diet ('Detox Diet') focuses on eating in a way that helps clear the body of toxins. The liver is the most important organ in this cleansing process because it is the body's natural filter that helps convert toxins into substances that can be easily discarded. Some diet gurus claim it is possible to rid the liver of toxins that have been lying stagnant for years by simply restricting oneself to organic, raw foods and drinking a lot of water to flush the system.

Toxins Stored In Fat

Some toxins cannot be broken down by the liver and are sent to the body's fat cells for storage.

To get rid of these toxins, fat stores must be broken down. This means a person needs to LOSE EXCESS BODY FAT to get rid of stored toxins. Avoiding fruit during a detox diet is one way to encourage the burning of fat (and releasing of toxins) instead of burning the more easily accessible sugar from fruit.

What About Hormones?

Are hormones a toxin? For those who suffer Pure Menstrual Migraine (migraines that occur around the time of a woman's period due to a drop in estrogen levels), the answer may be yes. I have found that the frequency of menstrual related migraines for me has decreased significantly since I began the Migraine Diet.

My assumption is that with fewer other (ingested) toxins to process, my body has an easier time managing the hormone stresses brought on by menstruation. The end result is a less stressed toxin-processing system and fewer migraines

Clearing The Toxins

I followed a three week Detox plan that seemed, at the time, to be very extreme. Anyone considering a detoxification diet should research a plan that is right for them and discuss it with a professional.

The purpose of the detox diet I followed was to return my body to its naturally, slightly alkaline state and set my body's acidity at 'neutral'. At this 'neutral' setting my digestive system would be better able to eliminate toxins and break down the acids in my body, both of which can lead to sluggish digestion and unwanted stress on the system.

The food focus was on low acid, raw foods that are nutritionally plentiful. By eating these foods, not only would I return my system to 'neutral', my palate would be altered and I would learn to appreciate the natural flavors of all foods. The diet recommended I cleanse the liver by eating raw vegetables such as broccoli, spinach and other dark green leafy veggies which contain vitamin B and minerals essential to healthy liver function. It encouraged the drinking of plenty of water (at least two liters a day) and suggested I be aware of detox 'symptoms' which could occur within two days of beginning the program. I did not experience these symptoms, though the release of toxins from the cleansing liver are purported to cause nausea, stomach pain, headaches and palpitations in some.

Addressing food addictions and cravings during the three week diet was an issue. My daily 'hit' of dark chocolate was not easy to give up but it was an accomplishment and an important part of being proactive in taking charge of my health. Shopping for locally grown, adequately ripened, organic, fresh foods was encouraged with emphasis on its nutritional value (based on where it is from, how far it has traveled and how long it has been stored).

The detox diet suggested the use of herbal preparations and vitamins during the three week program as a way to boost the effects of the diet. I avoided these items due to the prevalence of preservatives and additives in most supplements.

Foods To Avoid While On The Three Week Detox Diet

sugar, chocolate, candy, coffee, decaffeinated coffee, tea, cake, doughnuts, cookies, wheat, yeast, gluten, dairy products, red meat, fruit, alcohol, processed condiments or spreads like ketchup, mustard, vinegar, jam, jelly.

Foods that are Acid-Forming in the body were to be avoided during the detox although some (like chick peas) are also deemed excellent for liver health and were encouraged for everyday diet after detox.

Alkaline & Acidic Foods: Eat Alkaline, Avoid Acidic

Alkaline Foods

Vegetables: *Beets, Broccoli, Cabbage, Carrot, Cauliflower, Celery, Chard Greens, Collard Greens, Dandelion, Eggplant, Garlic, Green Beans, Green Peas, Kale, Kohlrabi , Lettuce, Mushrooms, Mustard Greens, Onions, Parsnips, Peppers, Pumpkin, Radishes, Rutabaga, Spinach, Sprouts, Sweet Potatoes, Tomatoes raw, Watercress, Wheat Grass*

Fruits: *Apple, Apricot, Avocado, Banana, Blackberries, Cantaloupe, Cherries, Coconut,*

Currants, Dates, Figs, Grapes, Grapefruit, Honeydew Melon, Lemon, Lime, Nectarine, Orange, Peach, Pear, Pineapple, Raisins, Raspberries, Rhubarb, Strawberries, Tangerine, Watermelon

Proteins: *Almonds, Chestnuts, Millet*

Sweeteners: *Stevia*

Spices: *Chili Pepper, Cinnamon, Curry, Ginger, Herbs, Miso, Mustard , Sea Salt*

Other: *Apple Cider, Vinegar, Bee Pollen, Mineral Water , Molasses, Probiotic Cultures*

Acidic Foods

Vegetables: *Corn, Olives, Winter Squash*

Fruits: *Blueberries, Canned Fruit, Cranberries, Currants , Plums, Prunes*

Grains: *Barley, Oat Bran, Wheat Bran, Bread, Corn, Cornstarch, Crackers, Flour, Hemp Seed, Macaroni, Oatmeal/Oats, Quinoa, Rice, Rye,*

Spelt, Wheat, Wheat Germ

Legumes & Beans: *Almond Milk, Black Beans, Chick Peas, Green Peas, Kidney Beans, Lentils, Pinto Beans, Red Beans, Rice Milk, Soy Beans, Soy Milk, White Beans*

Dairy: *All Dairy (except goat's milk), Butter , Cheese, Ice Cream/Ice Milk*

Nuts: *Cashews, Peanuts & Peanut Butter, Pecans, Tahini, Walnuts*

Animal Protein: *Beef, Chicken, Clams, Duck, Eggs, Fish, Goose, Lamb, Lobster, Mutton, Oyster, Pork Rabbit*

Sweeteners: *Carob, Corn Syrup, Sugar*

Alcohol: *Beer, Hard Liquor & Spirits, Wine*

Other: *Cocoa, Coffee, Ketchup & Mustard, Pepper, Soft Drinks, Vinegar*

Drugs *Aspirin, Tobacco*

*The foods indicated above are considered alkaline-forming or acid-forming *after* digestion. Their groupings have nothing to do with the pH of the food *before* it is eaten. A lemon for example, is a very acidic food before it has been consumed. However, after combining with digestive juices, the end product in the body is very alkaline.

Clearing The Toxins: Interesting Food Facts

Supporting information that I found useful on the road to better eating included some facts I gathered while researching detox diets. Notably, I discovered that many of the fruits we buy in the supermarket are picked far before they are ripe and are therefore acid-forming instead of alkaline when digested. Also, foods belonging to the Nightshade Family (including peppers, tomatoes, cucumbers, potatoes and aubergines) originate from the poison-ivy family and are known to cause food intolerances in some people.

If alcohol cannot be avoided on a night out (after a detox diet is complete), purer alcohols – vodka, gin or tequila - are the 'cleaner' choices. They are less harmful because they contain fewer chemical by-products of fermentation than wine, beer or champagne.

~

So, What's Left To Eat?

After the Detox Diet, I began to think about food beyond its taste and developed an interest in what the food was doing inside my body and *to* my body. As I cut out more and more additives & preservatives I began to wonder *are there any foods left for me to eat?*

As I stated earlier, **it is impossible to cut out all additives & preservatives from your diet and still have something to eat!** Avoiding foods that contain additives and preservatives has seriously limited the foods on my list of edibles but I have found a balance, and my menus now consist mostly of fresh vegetables and fruits (frozen fruits are also great), fresh fish and poultry, legumes, rice, nuts, vegetable oils, low yeast and unprocessed products, herbal teas and loads of plain water.

Homemade salsas, ketchup and ice cream are also big favorites. I avoid prepackaged produce and ensure all fresh items are well ventilated to avoid spoilage. When I purchase packaged food items, I always look for ingredient lists that are as short as possible; a short list of ingredients usually means less processing has taken place and fewer additives and preservatives have been used. Canned items often contain preserving agents and I use my discretion when deciding whether or not to take the risk.

Initially, when I stopped eating heavily flavored processed foods, I felt my meals had no taste. But when I began experimenting with herbs like basil, dill, sage, mustard, cumin, curry and others, and I began to taste the *food* not just the additives, I realized there was a whole world of taste outside the over-processed, too-salty options I had experienced until then.

~

Foods In My Cupboard: Ingredient Lists

Below are the ingredient lists of some of the foods in my cupboard. Note that not all are completely free of additives. Note also, how short the ingredient lists are. Additives and ingredients suspect as migraine triggers are highlighted in **bold** print.

Puffed Cereal/ Ingredients: whole hard red winter wheat, evaporated can juice, whole long grain brown rice, whole oats, whole barley, whole triticale, whole rye, whole buckwheat, honey, sesame seeds.

Oats/ Ingredients: 100% prairie grown oats

1% Yogurt/ Ingredients: **milk ingredients**, active bacterial cultures

Organic Peanut Butter/ Ingredients: organic peanuts, sea salt

Canned Tuna/ Ingredients: skipjack tuna, water, salt.

Canned Chick Peas/ Ingredients: chick peas, water, salt, **disodium EDTA**

Canned Tomatoes/ Ingredients: tomatoes, tomato juice, salt, **citric acid, calcium chloride**

Lentils/ Ingredients: red split lentils

Snack Crackers/ Ingredients: rice meal, safflower oil, salt.

Mixed Nuts/ Ingredients: cashews, almonds, pecans, hazelnuts, brazil nuts, vegetable oil (peanut and/or cottonseed and/or **soybean** and/or sunflower), salt

Imported Dark Chocolate/ Ingredients: cocoa mass, sugar, cocoa butter**, natural bourbon vanilla beans**, may contain traces of peanuts, hazelnuts, almonds, milk and **soya lecithin**.

Fresh Fruits & Vegetables/ Ingredients**:** fruits & vegetables

A few of my favorite, very flavorful recipes are described in the **Recipes** section at the end of this book.

~

The Glycemic Index

Most publications reference the Glycemic Index (G.I.) in relation to diabetes and weight loss but I have found it useful also, in controlling my migraines. G.I. research led me to recognize the important role highly processed and highly sugared foods play in our diets and our body functions. These foods cause spikes in blood-sugar levels which lead to unnecessary stresses on the body due to rapid system fluctuations and raised insulin levels.

The Glycemic Index measures the rate at which the body breaks down or digests foods and converts it into glucose for energy. The faster the food is digested, the higher its rating on the Index. Sugar, which is very quickly dissolved into the bloodstream, is given a rating of 100 on the Glycemic Index and all other foods are scored against that number. Foods that rate high on the Glycemic Index are often highly processed items such as packaged cookies and chips. These items, in their ready-to-eat state, have already been so processed the body is not required to work very hard to break them down. This means quick digestion, spiking blood sugar levels and unnecessary stress on the body.

Slowing the digestive process then, with *unprocessed*, slow release foods such as unrefined grains or old fashioned oatmeal will provide a more time-consuming challenge for the digestive system and energy (glucose sugars) will be released more slowly into the body. Various factors, including how foods are cooked and their fat and protein content can also affect the rate of digestion. Cooking can increase the G.I. rating of foods by swelling starch molecules, softening the food and making it faster to digest. Fat and protein content can slow the rate of stomach emptying so foods are digested at a slower rate.

Utilizing the Glycemic Index is an effective method for identifying slow glucose-release foods that will help maintain even blood sugar levels and avoid the stresses of rapid blood sugar fluctuations in the body. To further ensure stable blood sugar levels it is important to eat at regular times and never skip meals.

Glycemic Index: Foods & Their Ratings

Breads: White bread 71-77,   Wholemeal bread 69,   Pumpernickel 41-46,   Dark rye 76, Sourdough 57,   Heavy mixed grain 30-45

Pasta / Grains: Pasta cooked 'al-dente' 32-64, Chana dal 8,   Barley 25,   Bulgar 48,   Buckwheat 54,   Short Grain Rice 72,   Instant Rice 87

Legumes: Lentils 28,   Soybeans 18,   Baked beans (canned) 48

Potatoes: Boiled 56,   French Fries 75, Baked 93

Breakfast cereals: Cornflakes 84,   Rice Krispies 82,   Cheerios 83,   Puffed Wheat 80,   Bran flakes 74,   Bran Buds with psyllium 42,   All Bran 42, Porridge 46,   Oat Bran 50

Snack foods: Mars Bar 65,   Soda Crackers 74, Jelly beans 80,   Pretzels 89

Fruits: Apple 38,   Plum 39,   Orange 44, Peach 42 , Banana 55,   Watermelon 72

Dairy foods: Milk; full fat 27,   Milk; skim 32,   Ice-cream; full fat 61,   Yogurt; low fat with fruit 33

Soft and sports drinks: Fanta 68 ,   Gatorade 78

What About Aspartame?

*The Glycemic Index is all about cutting sugar from your diet, and aspartame is often suggested as a sugar substitute. It's important to note that aspartame is known as a potent migraine trigger because of the **excitotoxins** which form as it is digested.*

***Excitotoxins** are amino acids which cause nerve cells in the brain to fire spasmodically and cause an eventual burn out or damage of neural tissue.*

Other Factors That May Trigger Migraine

Other factors which have had a hand in reducing the severity and frequency of migraines for me have had to do with lifestyle choices. In particular, I have modified stress, sleep, exercise and household cleaning habits.

Stress

Stress is easy to overlook when considering what may or may not be the cause of migraines. My initial response when I was told I needed to 'manage the stress in my life' was bewilderment. Stress is *uncontrollable* I thought. Isn't that the whole point of its effectiveness? Stress hormones take over when our rational minds don't know what else to do and then we either 'fight' or 'take flight' from whatever is causing the stress.

But what I didn't consider was that the 'fight or flight' response to stress is not designed for modern day living. Most of our modern stressors are psychological (as opposed to physical) and involve relationships and life changes that create prolonged exposure to the ancient stress hormones our bodies produce. As a result, humans today may be running on the 'fight or flight' reaction longer than it's intended to operate and this overexposure to stress hormones can disrupt almost all of the body's processes. If the 'fight or flight' response never shuts off, stress hormones can lead to depression, anxiety, and sleep & personality disorders.

Studies also suggest that chronic activation of stress hormones may alter the operation and structure of brain cells that are critical for memory formation and function. With this information in mind it is difficult to overlook the importance of managing stress in the quest to manage migraines. I have often noted 'stressful' events which begin one to two weeks prior to a migraine and find that when I allow them to take over my world (I become agitated, tense, shaky, weepy, over-stimulated, exhausted, unable to sleep, overwhelmed, out-of-control), the migraine follows shortly thereafter. The best way for me to reduce the feelings of stress in my life is to simply STOP for one day. The kids, the business and the mess can manage for one day without my immediate and constant attention.

Slowing Down When Over-Stimulated

- breathe deeply
- turn off the noise (tv/computer/radio/lights)
- relax the jaw, tongue, neck, top and back of head /

close your eyes

- say no to unnecessary commitments or requests

- sit and do nothing for 30 minutes (really! do nothing, just listen to yourself breathe)

- write down what is causing anxiety

-take considered action to getting rid of stressors causing anxiety

- take a nap

- admit you've had enough and go to bed for the night

-learn about meditation and do it! (every day)

Sleep

We live in a culture that very often tells us that asking for or getting too much sleep means we are lazy. A nap is a sure sign of 'too much time on our hands' or 'too little to do' in the day. In my experience, if I suggest I am tired by 9.00 p.m., my comments are often greeted by a chorus of concerned voices regarding fatigue as a sign of mental depression. But here is what I have learned: I am not lazy and I am not depressed. My body just happens to function differently than (perhaps) a large percentage of the population and I need a lot of sleep. I am not willing to feel awful all day due to a lack of sleep and I know that I MUST get the sleep I need to avoid migraines and feel my best.

Exhaustion is often cited as a precursor to migraine attacks. Why is this? Scientists are unsure why we need sleep. Studies have shown that sleep is an essential part of maintaining normal levels of cognitive skills such as speech, memory and flexible thinking. Energy supplies are restored and muscle tissue is rebuilt throughout the body as we pass through the various cycles of sleep.

Some research has suggested our brain cells reset their sodium & potassium ratios when the brain is mentally 'disengaged', just before we fall asleep. Lack of sleep can seriously affect our brain's ability to function, making us irritable, forgetful, unfocused and groggy. According to 'The science of sleep' at bbc.co.uk, 17 hours of sustained wakefulness leads to a decrease in performance equivalent to a blood alcohol level of 0.05% (two glasses of wine).

Exercise

When people talk about exercise, I usually hear one of two things: 1) I don't have time to exercise or 2) I exercise and I exercise hard because that's the best way to get in shape (the 'no pain, no gain' theory).

I can understand both points of view but have found that neither is helpful in managing my migraines or my health. *Moderation* is the key. Moderation allows for short periods of exercise on a regular schedule, with minimal head movement (commonly known to bring on migraine) and does not require gym memberships and fancy equipment. It allows me to strengthen my whole body so I am better equipped to deal with a migraine and helps me avoid the toxins that are produced in my body during heavy exercise (see following, "*Toxins During Exercise*").

Additionally, I have noticed that if I exercise too hard or for too long I become so hungry I eat with abandon and discover two hours later that I have made bad food choices. My moderate exercise routine is simple: I *walk* at least 20-40 minutes a day. This does not mean I put on jogging clothes and running shoes and drive out to the track. I walk around the block, or down the street. On an extremely busy day I will park far away from the grocery store and make the walk across the parking lot. Sometimes the recommended "20-45 minutes" of exercise per day seems like too much of a commitment. But I believe there is more benefit in exercising for a short time (less than the recommendation) than not at all.

In addition to walking, I take ten minutes to do yoga or pilates and stretching five mornings a week. These exercises, which employ the use of the whole body, are strengthening and toning in a manner isolating workouts have never been for me. There is no need to push hard and 'feel the burn'. If I stray from this routine of moderation in exercise and I workout until my muscles burn and my body is exhausted, I always (always) suffer a migraine one to two days later.

Toxins During Exercise: Could They Trigger Migraine?

During intense exercise, various chemical compounds in the body become imbalanced.

*Of the many changes that occur during intense exercise, **acidosis** (which is a drop in arterial pH below 7.35) or abnormally high concentrations of **lactic acid (lactate**) in the blood can occur.*

*As **lactate** is formed during a process of fermentation (a process commonly linked to migraine,) and both acidosis **and** high lactate concentrations represent imbalanced and irregular conditions for the body's chemistry, is it possible that they may be migraine triggers?*

Hydration

Our bodies are made up of 75 % water and it is essential to the healthy functioning of all our body systems. A shortage of water slows the release of toxins and waste products from our body making us more susceptible to migraines, headache and fatigue.

I start my day with a large glass of water and drink another glass every 1 ½ hours. I avoid flavored waters because of the excessive amounts of additives and flavorings.

Cleaning Products

Cleaning products are hard to pin down as specific migraine triggers, but what I do know is that most are highly toxic and leave me feeling disoriented and sick after use.

I buy non-toxic products whenever possible and avoid unnecessary fragrance sprays and mists.

Medication Specific To Migraine

The use of medication specific to migraine is an important part of The Migraine Diet. I began my diet research because of the lack of success I was experiencing with prescription medications but have not ceased in my search for pharmaceutical solutions.

I believe in covering as many bases as possible in attempting to free myself of migraines and am currently following the Migraine Diet and utilizing prophylactic medication to control migraines.

~

What Does It All Mean?

After all this, I have seen the affect food and lifestyle can have on my health.

Altering my diet and lifestyle to avoid toxins has brought a decrease in the frequency and severity of migraines for me and I have begun to see possible links to how excess toxins may be short-circuiting my brain and making me sick with migraines.

I have seen the complexity of migraine and the promise of current research in finding better migraine management solutions. I have experienced an increase in energy, improved sleep and sleep patterns, loss of body fat and consistently maintained lowered body weight for over four years (and counting) through diet, moderate exercise and a commitment to cutting additives and other toxins from my diet. I have made a conscious effort to reduce fat intake to avoid storing unwanted toxins in the fat cells of my body and have found benefit in avoiding diet foods and unnecessary medications & supplements and their toxic additives and fillers.

I look forward to learning more about healthy living and wish health and success to all who read this book.

Recipes

The following recipes may not be for everyone as some may contain ingredients that are on your personal 'trigger list'. If this is the case, experiment with the recipe and try substituting non-trigger foods for those that cause trouble.

Black Bean Dip

1 red bell pepper
¾ cup minced fresh cilantro (one bunch)
3 tablespoons chopped green onion

2 tablespoons lime juice

2 tablespoons balsamic vinegar

2 tablespoons hot sauce

½ teaspoon ground allspice

½ teaspoon ground cumin

¼ teaspoon salt

¼ teaspoon black pepper

30 ounces canned black beans, drained & well rinsed

1 jalapeño pepper, seeded and diced

1 garlic clove, minced

chopped red pepper (optional)

Cut bell peppers in half lengthwise, discarding seeds and membranes. Place pepper halves, skin side up, on a foil-lined baking sheet and flatten. Broil 5 minutes or until blackened. Place blackened pepper in a sealed container, let stand 5 minutes, then peel. Place pepper and the following 12 ingredients in a food processor and process until smooth. Spoon into bowl and garnish with chopped bell pepper.

Strawberry Spinach Salad

In a large salad bowl mix:

3 large bunches spinach, rinsed & dried

1 head romaine, rinsed & dried

Make Dressing:

½ cup vegetable oil

1/3 cup white vinegar

2-3 tablespoons maple syrup

1 tablespoon dijon mustard

½ teaspoon salt

1 small red onion, finely chopped

Just before serving, dress the spinach and romaine then add:

1 pint fresh strawberries, sliced

2/3 cup sunflower seeds, salted

toss lightly

Bean And Chickpea Salad

Mix in large bowl:

1 can black beans, drained & rinsed

1 can chick peas, drained & rinsed

1 can kernel corn, drained (optional, depending on your sensitivity to corn products)

add 2 medium carrots, chopped

1 broccoli floret, cut into small pieces

½ roasted red pepper, chopped

5 pieces sundried tomato (in oil), chopped

Mix well with dried or fresh basil, dill, oregano, black pepper, sea salt,

Dress with:

1/3 cup balsamic vinegar

½ cup olive oil

1 tablespoon fresh lemon juice.

Garnish with sunflower seeds or nuts and eat as is or with greens.

Curried Lentils

1 tablespoon olive oil

1 very small onion, minced

2 medium carrots, chopped

2 cloves garlic, minced

1 cup dried red lentils

2 cups chicken stock (recipe to follow)

1 cup water

½ teaspoon chopped gingerroot

1-2 teaspoons curry powder

3 ribs celery, finely chopped

3 tablespoons balsamic vinegar

plain yogurt as garnish

Combine olive oil, onion, carrot and garlic in a large microwave safe bowl. Microwave on High for 3 minutes. Add lentils, chicken stock, water and gingerroot. Cover with a vented lid. Microwave on High 25 minutes, stirring once. Stir in curry powder, celery, balsamic. Serve with yogurt and pita chips.

Chicken Stock

Combine in a large stock pot:

whole chicken, cooked with meat removed

drippings from cooked chicken

1 bunch celery, chopped into 2 inch pieces

5 medium carrots, chopped into 2 inch pieces

5 parsnips, chopped into 2 inch pieces

2 large onions, chopped into large chunks

1 leek, cleaned well, white parts chopped into large

chunks

1 head garlic, peeled and chopped

1 teaspoon salt

whole peppercorns

dill weed (fresh or dried)

basil (fresh or dried)

oregano (fresh or dried)

sage (fresh or dried)

marjoram (fresh or dried)

Add water to 2" from top, cover and heat on medium (do not boil or the stock will become cloudy)

Reduce heat and simmer at least 2 hours. Cool stock in refrigerator overnight. Skim fat off cooled stock and strain using cheese cloth.

Soup can be frozen in small batches or used immediately.

Thick Peanut Soup

2 cups chopped onions

1 tablespoon peanut or vegetable oil

½ teaspoon cayenne

1 teaspoon grated peeled fresh gingerroot

1 cup chopped carrots

2 cups chopped sweet potatoes (up to 1 cup white potatoes can be substituted)

4 cups chicken stock or vegetable stock or water

2 cups tomato juice

1 cup natural peanut butter

1 tablespoon sugar (optional)

½ cup chopped scallions or chives

Sauté onions in oil until translucent. Stir in cayenne, gingerroot & carrots and sauté 2 minutes. Mix in potatoes & stock and bring soup to a boil then simmer 15 min. In a blender/food processor, puree the vegetables with the cooking liquid & tomato juice. Return puree to soup pot. Stir in peanut butter until smooth. Add sugar to taste. Serve with plenty of chopped scallions or chives.

Almond Fish

4 filets boneless white fish

1 egg

1/2 cup milk

1/2 cup almond meal (also called almond flour)

1/2 cup rice flour

1 tablespoon baking powder

1/2 teaspoon salt

1/4 teaspoon each dill & parsley

1-3 tablespoons butter or vegetable oil

lemon wedges

Rinse the fish.

Whisk the egg and milk together in a small bowl and put all pieces of fish in the mix. It can sit while you complete the next step.

In a flat dish with sides (a square baking dish is good), mix the almond meal, rice flour, baking powder, salt, dill and parsley.

Take one piece of fish from the milk & egg mix and place in the flour mixture. Coat both sides, pressing lightly on the fish to get the flour to stick. When both sides are coated, carefully place the fish on a clean plate. Coat all pieces.

Heat a large frying pan with the butter or vegetable

oil to hot (medium high) and gently lay the fish in the pan. Lower heat to medium.

Cook until browned (about 2-3 minutes) and flip the filets; you may need to add extra oil before flipping if all the oil has all been absorbed.

Cook another 2-3 minutes.

Serve with vegetables and rice or potatoes and a squeeze of lemon.

Frozen Strawberry Cream (no milk)

Get out your ice-cream maker for this frozen dessert. Minimal ingredients and *so* tasty!

2 cups frozen strawberries, thawed
1/2 cup sugar

Using a hand blender, blend the strawberries until puréed. Pour into a small pot and add sugar. Bring to a boil on the stove, then cool in the fridge while assembling and mixing the following ingredients,

2 - 400 ml cans organic full fat coconut milk (look for a brand without thickeners and additives)
1/4 cup sugar

1/2 teaspoons ground vanilla bean

Using the hand blender, blend the coconut milk, sugar and vanilla until creamy. Cover and put in the fridge for 2 hours.

After 2 hours, blend the coconut cream again to add air into the mix and pour into the ice cream maker as per manufacturer's instructions.

Add 1/2 to 3/4 of the purée while the coconut cream mixes and continue to mix until it is ice-creamy.

Pour the creamy mix into a glass 9" square cake pan and drizzle the remaining purée on top. Using a knife, marble the purée into the creamy mix. Cover and freeze.

This dessert will freeze very hard and is tastiest when allowed to thaw for 10-15 minutes on the counter . Cut into squares using a heated knife and serve with extra fruit.

Morning Shake Pear, Papaya, Pineapple

1 pear, cut in chunks

1/2 cup frozen or fresh papaya

1/2 cup frozen or fresh pineapple

1 tsp. coconut oil

1/2 cup water

3/4 to 1 cup coconut water

Put all ingredients in a blender and mix on high until very smooth. Use a big straw! Add ice if desired.

Morning Shake RAW

1/2 avocado

1 pear or apple, cut in chunks

1 stalk celery, cut in chunks

juice of 1/2 lemon

1 beet leaf

1 tsp chia seeds

1-2 cups water or to taste

Put all ingredients in a blender and mix on high until very smooth. Use a big straw!

Good luck and good health!

Let me know how you're doing.

info@themigrainediet.com

References

Publications Buchholz, David. Heal Your Headache: *The 1 2 3 Program*. New York, NY: Workman Publishing Company, Inc, 2002.Burks, Susan L. Managing Your Migraine: *A Migraine Sufferer's Practical Guide*. Totowa, New Jersey: Humana Press Inc., 1994.Gallop, Rick. The Glycemic Index Diet: *The Easy, Healthy way to Permanent Weight Loss*. Canada: Random House Canada, 2002.Mindell, Earl. Unsafe at Any Meal: *How to Avoid Hidden Toxins in Your Food*. New York, NY: The McGraw-Hill Companies, 2002.South, Valerie. Migraine. Toronto, Canada: Key Porter Books Limited, 2001.Winter, Ruth. A Consumer's Dictionary of Food Additives*: Descriptions in Plain English of More Than 12,000 Ingredients both Harmful and Desirable Found in Foods*. 6th Edition. New York, N.Y.: Three Rivers Press, 2004.**Online**BBC –

Science & Nature – Human Body and Mind – What is sleep "http://www.bbc.co.uk" www.bbc.co.uk

National Institute of Neurological Disorders and Stroke,

"http://www.ninds.nih.gov/disorders/migraine/migraine.htm"

http://www.ninds.nih.gov/disorders/migraine/migraine.htm

"http://www.healthyweightforum.org/eng/articles/glycemic-index/"

http://www.healthyweightforum.org/eng/articles/glycemic-index/

"http://home.bluegrass.net/~jclark/alkaline_foods.htm"

http://home.bluegrass.net/~jclark/alkaline_foods.htm

"http://www.migrainesolutions.com/migraine_resources/migraine_glossary.html"

http://www.migrainesolutions.com/migraine_resources/migraine_glossary.html

"http://www.msgmyth.com/hidename.htm"

http://www.msgmyth.com/hidename.htm

"http://professionals.epilepsy.com/page/glossary.html#m"

http://professionals.epilepsy.com/page/glossary.html#m   "http://www.wikipedia.org/"

http://www.wikipedia.org/ National Institute of Neurological Disorders and Stroke, HYPERLINK "http://www.ninds.nih.gov/disorders/migraine/migraine.htm"

http://www.ninds.nih.gov/disorders/migraine/migraine.htmWikipedia, Online Encyclopedia. HYPERLINK "http://en.wikipedia.org/wiki/Excitotoxicity"

http://en.wikipedia.org/wiki/Excitotoxicity U.S. Food and Drug Administration, U.S. Dept. of Health and Human Services.

"http://www.fda.gov/oc/opacom/fda101/sld001.html"

http://www.fda.gov/oc/opacom/fda101/sld001.htmlG RAS (Generally Recognized as Safe) Food Ingredients: Nitrates and Nitrites (Including Nitrosamines)," 1972. (report prepared for the U.S. Food and Drug Administration (FDA) by Battele-Columbus Laboratories and Department of Commerce, Springfield, VA 22151) Stress: unhealthy response to the pressures of life, MayoClinic.com, by Mayo Clinic Staff, Sept 12, 2006.

" ALL DISEASE
BEGINS
IN THE GUT. "

-HIPPOCRATES

Printed in Great Britain
by Amazon